Cooking Clean

Practical Food Safety for Every Kitchen

A Guide from How2Conquer

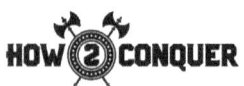

Published by How2Conquer
Atlanta, Georgia
www.how2conquer.com

How2Conquer is an imprint of White Deer Publishing, LLC
www.whitedeerpublications.com

© 2023 by How2Conquer

All rights reserved. No part of this publication may be reproduced, stored in a retrieval system, or transmitted in any form or by any means — for example, electronic, photocopy, recording — without the prior written permission of the publisher. The only exception is brief quotations in printed reviews.

Illustrations and cover design by Telia Garner
Book interior design by Charlotte Bleau
Edited by Katherine Guntner and Emily Owens

Library of Congress Cataloging-in-Publication Data is on file at the Library of Congress, Washington, DC.

Print ISBN 978-1-945783-09-8
Ebook ISBN 978-1-945783-10-4

Contents

Introduction 1
About Food Safety 2
Common Symptoms of Food Poisoning 2
About Terminology 3
Cleaning vs. Sanitizing vs. Disinfecting 3
Understanding Chemicals for Food Safety 5
How Food Becomes Unsafe 9

Six Steps to Cooking Clean 11
1. Good Personal Hygiene 12
Good Kitchen Hygiene 12
2. Avoid Cross-Contamination and Keep a Sanitized Kitchen 14
Avoiding Cross-Contamination 14
Handwashing Dishes, Pots, Pans, and Cooking Utensils .. 15
Sanitizing Countertops and Other Surfaces 16
3. Treat Your Food Right 18
Potentially Hazardous Foods 18
Temperature Management 18
4. Manage Your Pantry 23
Dry Goods Management 23
5. "Is This Still Good?" 27
6. Recalled Food Product 30
Handle Recalled Food Product 30

Top Tips for Cooking Clean 33

Wrap Up & Resources 35
Resources 36

About the Expert 37
    Michelle Newcome 37
About How2Conquer Guides 38

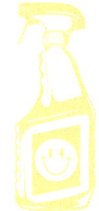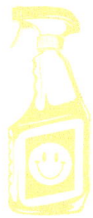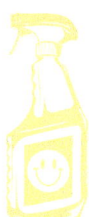

Introduction

If you aren't used to cooking at home, it can feel a bit overwhelming to throw in complex food safety rules, but keeping your food and family safe doesn't have to be a Michelin star production. We've collected some basics for you in this booklet, and we hope they'll help give you a good feeling of control over the safety of the food you're cooking for yourself and your family.

Food is a tremendous source of nurturing and comfort. If you're on a journey to cook at home more (or you've been a home cook for a long time) this simple guide will help you avoid the risk of unintended food contamination.

In addition to an increase in home cooking, rising food prices mean we're being more careful about food waste, which makes how you store food critically important.

We'll introduce some basics before we get into the nitty gritty of how to maintain your kitchen while *Cooking Clean*.

About Food Safety

Food safety is about keeping you and your family from becoming sick. No one likes an upset tummy after eating home cooking.

Restaurants and commercial kitchens follow a set of guidelines called HACCP (Hazard Analysis and Critical Control Points). These guidelines were developed by NASA to keep astronauts safely fed in space. HACCP is the core of most food safety codes in the US. You don't need to go as far as HACCP standards in your home kitchen, but we've adapted some of its common measures to help keep your home kitchen safe for your family.

A FOODBORNE ILLNESS is a disease that is carried or transmitted to people by food. Most foodborne illnesses are caused by microorganisms such as bacteria, viruses, parasites, and fungi.

Once harmful microorganisms have been transmitted onto food, they can grow rapidly, especially in high-protein food and low-acid conditions or when high moisture is present.

The Centers for Disease Control and Prevention (CDC) estimates that each year 48 million people in the United States get sick from a foodborne illness. Of those, 128,000 require hospitalization and 3,000 die.

Common Symptoms of Food Poisoning

Nausea, vomiting, stomach cramps, and diarrhea are all symptoms of a foodborne illness. Symptoms can range from mild to catastrophic.

About Terminology

Cleaning vs. Sanitizing vs. Disinfecting

We tend to use these terms interchangeably, but they're distinctly different procedures with different purposes. It helps to understand the purpose of each as the first step in food safety.

 Specific chemicals for sanitizing and disinfecting state on the label which microorganisms they kill.

CLEANER: A PRODUCT THAT REMOVES DIRT AND SOIL

- Cleaners are used on a number of surfaces.
- Cleaning is the process of removing visible debris.

And now it gets more complicated.

SANITIZER: AN AGENT THAT REDUCES DISEASE-CAUSING BACTERIA ON FOOD-CONTACT SURFACES

- Sanitizers are used on countertops, flatware, food, glasses, pans, plates, pots, preparation equipment, trays, utensils, etc.
- Because sanitizers are meant for use on food preparation surfaces, they're tested against the most common bacteria that cause foodborne illness (*staphylococcus*, *E. coli*, *salmonella*, etc.) because if they can kill those bacteria, they're strong enough to kill many others.
- Generally, a sanitizer kills 99.999 percent of specific bacteria when used correctly.

DISINFECTANT: AN AGENT THAT REDUCES INFECTION ON NONPOROUS SURFACES BY DESTROYING MICROORGANISMS

- Disinfectants are used on bathtubs, bed frames, ceilings, chairs, floors, sinks, showers, toilets, walls, etc.
- Disinfectants have a 100 percent kill rate on certain microorganisms, but not all. For example, they're not 100 percent effective against bacterial spores.
- This is why most food safety refers to SANITIZER and SANITIZATION — because the cause of most foodborne illness is bacteria.
- Disinfectants must be tested extensively and list everything they kill on the label.

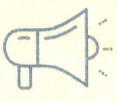

SANITIZING is for killing bacteria that cause foodborne illness, but for a virus, you have to take different steps and use a DISINFECTANT. See "2. Avoid Cross-Contamination and Keep a Sanitized Kitchen" on page 14.

Sanitizing and disinfecting chemicals are not designed for human consumption. DO NOT ingest, inject, or otherwise use these chemicals on or in your body.

Introduction

Understanding Chemicals for Food Safety

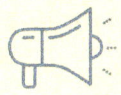
See "About Terminology" on page 3 for more notes on the difference between cleaning, sanitizing, and disinfecting.

Household bleach acts against most microorganisms, including bacteria, which is why it can be used as both a sanitizer AND a disinfectant depending on the concentration.

DO NOT use bleach that is designated "splashless" or "cling," as it has a different chemical makeup and additives. Also, DO NOT use scented bleach — that's only for laundry. Use ONLY regular bleach on home surfaces.

Bleach brands can vary greatly in the amount or concentration of active chemicals (such as sodium hypochlorite). The ratios listed in the table on page 7 are for standard Clorox bleach. Always read the label of your bleach for the correct ratios.

1. UNDERSTAND THE PURPOSE OF CHEMICALS
    - The goals of cleaning the kitchen and items you use are to: remove what you can see (food and dirt) and sanitize what you can't see (microorganisms such as bacteria and viruses).
    - Cleaning removes visible signs of soil and debris while sanitizing with chemicals removes harmful levels of bacterial contamination.

- In order to clean sufficiently to prevent contamination and foodborne illness, you must use products specifically designed for this purpose.
- For basic cleaning, hand soap for handwashing and dish soap for dishwashing work beautifully. For cleaning counters and surfaces, you can use a specific kitchen product.
- For sanitizing, you need something more specific and typically chemical-based.

REMEMBER: we're more concerned with SANITIZING when it comes to food preparation and kitchens. DISINFECTING is for bathrooms and changing tables.

2. EXERCISE GREAT CARE WITH CHEMICALS

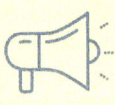

Be very careful with any kind of chemical, even one that is typically marketed or sold for use in the home.

- Only use chemicals in well-ventilated areas.
- Wear gloves to protect your skin from exposure.
- Only mix bleach with cool water.
- Add the bleach to the water, not the water to the bleach.
- Label all bottles and containers that contain a sanitizing solution. Do not reuse bottles that have contained a sanitizing solution.
- Store any sanitizing solution well out of the reach of children.

Sanitizing Solution

Use on food contact surfaces like dishes, eating utensils, knives, pans, and pots (if you don't have a dishwasher). This represents approximately 100 ppm (parts per million).

Water	Bleach (strength 2.75%)	Bleach (strength 5.25–6.25%)	Bleach (strength 8.25%)
1 gallon (128 oz)	1 tablespoon	2 teaspoons	1 teaspoon
1 quart (32 oz) *typical spray bottle size*	1 teaspoon	½ teaspoon	¼ teaspoon

Disinfecting Solution

Use on bathrooms, countertops, door handles, light switches, and toilet seats — basically any nonporous and non-food contact surfaces. This represents approximately 600–800 ppm.

Water	Bleach (strength 2.75%)	Bleach (strength 5.25–6.25%)	Bleach (strength 8.25%)
1 gallon (128 oz)	⅓ cup plus 1 tablespoon	3 tablespoons	2 tablespoons
1 quart (32 oz) *typical spray bottle size*	1 ½ tablespoons	2 ¼ teaspoons	1 ½ teaspoons

- You can use commercial sanitizing products on counters and surfaces, but DO NOT USE COMMERCIAL SANITIZERS ON DISHES, PANS, POTS, OR UTENSILS unless the product is specifically designated for food surfaces and food contact.

DO NOT mix chemicals!

- Bleach + ammonia = toxic chloramine vapor
- Bleach + rubbing alcohol = toxic chloroform
- Bleach + vinegar = toxic chlorine gas
- Vinegar + peroxide = paracetic acid

3. KEEP ALL COUNTERS AND CUTTING BOARDS SANITIZED

Doing so means they'll be ready to use when you begin cooking. If you aren't sure about the level of cleanliness when you begin, start by sanitizing.

Put some of the sanitizing solution in a spray bottle for use on countertops and other surfaces. You can use commercial sanitizing wipes, but they honestly don't work as well as the sanitizing solution.

How Food Becomes Unsafe

1. **POOR PERSONAL HYGIENE**

   Examples of poor hygiene in the kitchen include not washing hands properly, not covering cuts, touching body parts, and wearing jewelry while cooking. Not controlling personal hygiene increases the risk of transmitting human-borne pathogens into food.

2. **CROSS-CONTAMINATION AND IMPROPER CLEANING AND SANITIZING**

   Cross-contamination describes the transfer of micro-organisms from one food or surface to another.

   Cross-contamination is caused by not washing hands, improper cleaning and sanitizing, surfaces and utensils touching both raw and ready-to-eat foods, and improperly storing raw foods above ready-to-eat foods.

   Foods are contaminated when they come into contact with surfaces that aren't cleaned and sanitized regularly.

3. **TIME-TEMPERATURE ABUSE AND IMPROPER FOOD STORAGE**

   Food that's allowed to remain in the temperature danger zone (40–140°F) can become potentially hazardous by allowing bacteria to multiply. Keeping hot foods hot and cold foods cold can prevent time-temperature abuse.

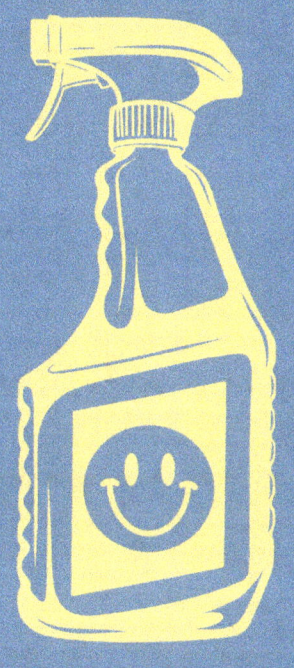

Six Steps to Cooking Clean

1. Good Personal Hygiene

You are the first step in food safety

The practices you put in place to control the spread of bacteria and human-borne microorganisms are critical to ruling a safe kitchen.

Good Kitchen Hygiene

1. THOROUGHLY WASH YOUR HANDS

    Wash your hands with soap and warm water before preparing food and at intervals during preparation (after handling raw meat, between steps, after you've touched the refrigerator handle, etc.).

    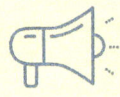 Always wash your hands after you've touched your phone. Phones are huge sources of contamination.

2. TAKE OFF YOUR JEWELRY

    Rings especially can harbor bacteria, but so can watches and bracelets.

3. COVER ALL CUTS WITH WATERPROOF DRESSINGS OR GLOVES

    Restaurant workers use brightly covered bandages in case they fall off and end up in prepared food.

4. TIE BACK LONG HAIR

    Hair isn't really a problem for food contamination, it's just pretty gross to get hair in your food — even when it's your own hair.

5. **DON'T PREPARE FOOD IF YOU'RE SICK**

   There's a pretty good chance you can transmit disease if you're sick since many diseases are transmitted via respiratory droplets, which can fall on food you're preparing.

6. **TASTE FOOD THE RIGHT WAY**

   Place a small amount into a separate container. Use a teaspoon to dip into the separate container to taste the food. Immediately wash the teaspoon and your hands.

2. Avoid Cross-Contamination and Keep a Sanitized Kitchen

Two words: clean and sanitize

We all grew up knowing kitchen cleanliness is important, but not everyone got the step-by-step instructions on what cleanliness ACTUALLY looks like. We hope these steps help.

 The goal of cleaning the kitchen and items you use: remove what you can see (food and dirt) and sanitize what you can't see (micro-organisms such as bacteria and viruses).

If you use a dishwasher, it takes care of the sanitizing for you via high heat and detergent. If you don't have a dishwasher, you'll need to work a bit harder at cleaning and sanitizing.

Avoiding Cross-Contamination

1. START AT THE GROCERY STORE
    - Separate proteins such as raw meat, poultry, seafood, eggs, and dairy from other foods in your cart.
    - At check out, be sure raw meat, poultry, and seafood are in separate bags to keep their juices away from other foods.

2. KEEP SEPARATE CUTTING BOARDS
    - Have a cutting board each for handling raw proteins, produce, and cooked foods.
    - The one you use for proteins should be a food-safe plastic cutting board because they're easier to clean with sanitizing solution.

- Don't forget to sanitize knives and other implements used to cut or handle raw foods.

3. CONTROL SPILLS

   - Clean up all spills immediately.
   - If a spill is from a potentially hazardous food (i.e. a protein), then use a disposable paper towel and throw it away immediately.

A surface has to be CLEAN before it can be SANITIZED. These are two separate steps.

Handwashing Dishes, Pots, Pans, and Cooking Utensils

1. REMOVE AS MUCH FOOD DEBRIS AS POSSIBLE
2. WASH IN HOT, SOAPY WATER

   Use a dishcloth you replace each day. Try to avoid sponges, as they can harbor microorganisms.

3. RINSE THOROUGHLY IN HOT WATER

   Leaving any soap residue has two risks: left soap can cause tummy troubles, and it makes it harder for the sanitizer to work.

4. SANITIZE WITH A BLEACH SOLUTION OR WITH HOT WATER

   - If you're using hot water, then it has to be REALLY HOT, and you need to submerge the dishes. If you're not food writer Nigella Lawson with her "asbestos hands," you should wear gloves.
   - You may be tempted to skip this step, but if you're concerned about contamination, have tiny children, or

care for an immunocompromised person, you'll want to do this added work.
- To effectively kill bacterial activity, you must soak items in the santizing solution for two minutes.
- If you're using the ratio for sanitizing solution (see "Sanitizing Solution" on page 7), there's no need to rinse after sanitizing.

5. ALLOW DISHES TO AIR DRY OR USE A CLEAN TEA TOWEL

By clean, we mean straight out of the stack of towels that've been washed in hot water and bleach.

Sanitizing Countertops and Other Surfaces

1. WIPE OFF CRUMBS, FOOD, OR ANY LOOSE DEBRIS

Using a dry towel, sweep it into your hand or a dust pan, and then throw it in the trash (the debris, not the dust pan).

2. WASH DOWN WITH A CLEAN DISHCLOTH THAT'S BEEN DIPPED IN HOT SOAPY WATER AND WRUNG OUT SLIGHTLY

In other words, no need to soak the entire kitchen.

3. SPRAY DOWN THE SURFACE WITH SANITIZING SOLUTION

If you're concerned about viruses — as during a pandemic or when taking care of someone sick — use the ratio listed for disinfection for countertops and other hard surfaces (see "Sanitizing Solution" on page 7).

Be careful about brushing up against counters that have been sprayed with bleach. Even a diluted solution can bleach your clothing and disintegrate natural fibers.

4. ALLOW TO AIR DRY

The solution needs to sit on the surface for a minimum of five minutes. If you want shiny surfaces, then go back over them with a clean and DRY towel after the five minutes or once they're dry.

5. GIVE YOUR SINK SOME EXTRA LOVE

Once your kitchen is clean at night, fill your sink with hot water and put in a capful of bleach. Leave overnight. Your sink will be sanitized and sparkling clean in the morning.

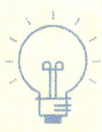

Run your dishwasher each night, even if it's not 100 percent full. This ensures dishes with food debris aren't sitting overnight creating bacteria growth.

3. Treat Your Food Right

Avoid time-temperature abuses and improper food storage

Potentially Hazardous Foods

You should be cautious with all foods, but there are three types of food that require especially careful management.

Potentially Hazardous Foods (PHFs) are foods that provide the ideal environment for bacteria to grow. PHFs are:

- High in protein
- High in moisture
- Low in acidity

Beans, chicken, dairy, pasta, rice, steak, etc., are all PHFs that, if not handled correctly, could cause serious illness. That's why it's so important that you're extremely careful in the way you handle food in order to control bacterial growth and prevent cross-contamination.

Temperature Management

1. KEEP UP WITH YOUR FRIDGE TEMPERATURE

    - The temperature inside should always be below 40°F (40°F-37°F is ideal). Use a thermometer to check. You can buy thermometers specifically designed for refrigerators.
    - Refrigerate or freeze meat and poultry the minute you're home from the store.
    - Keep the fridge door closed as much as possible, and don't store perishable items like milk or eggs in the door.
    - Stage your fridge so proteins (meat, poultry, and seafood) are always in the lowest drawer. Raw protein

often drips, and those spills have a high chance of creating cross-contamination.

2. THAW CORRECTLY

- Frozen foods are susceptible to contamination if improperly thawed.
- Freezing prevents bacteria from multiplying but doesn't kill it. Bacteria can and will multiply as food begins to thaw.
- Provide for free circulation of air between thawing foods to speed thawing.

 NEVER thaw food at room temperature.

- Thaw food in the refrigerator at 41°F or less.
- Thaw food by submerging it under running, drinkable water that is 70°F or less. It must be closely supervised.
- Thaw food as part of the cooking process.
- Thaw food in the microwave only if the food will be cooked immediately.

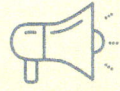 Watch supplies closely to avoid the need to thaw food quickly.

3. COOK IT UP RIGHT

- Know the minimum internal cooking temperatures required for various foods.
- Food (raw and cooked) can become unsafe if it dwells anywhere between 40°F and 140°F (time-

temperature abuse). Keep your fridge set to 37°F and make sure your cooked food hits above 140°F.

WATCH OUT FOR THE 100 DEGREES OF DOOM: anywhere between 40°F and 140°F.

Internal Meat Temperature Doneness

140°F	Rare beef, ham (precooked)
145°F	Medium rare beef, lamb
160°F	Medium beef, ham, lamb, veal (raw)
170°F	Well-done beef, lamb, pork, veal
180°F	Chicken and turkey (whole)

4. COOL RESPONSIBLY

- Cooling food to below 40°F slows bacteria growth. Freezing stops most bacteria growth, but allows many bacteria to survive.

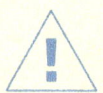

DO NOT cool large batches of food by simple refrigeration in stock pots, bains-marie, or any large, deep containers. Refrigerators are not capable of cooling such quantities through the danger zone rapidly enough.

- Divide large batches into smaller, shallow (no more than four inches deep) containers.
- For rapid cooling, immerse containers in an ice water bath (being careful not to allow any water to get into the container and possibly contaminate the food) and promptly refrigerate.

5. MANAGE YOUR LEFTOVERS

- Remember the two-hour rule for refrigeration. Perishable leftovers from a meal should not stay out of refrigeration for more than two hours.
- In hot weather (90°F or above) this time is reduced to one hour.

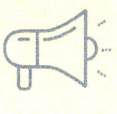

> Rice (and beans) are a primary culprit of a toxin-producing bacteria called *Bacillus cereus*. Exercise care with these foods to ensure they aren't left at room temperature for long periods.

- Divide leftovers into small portions and store in shallow, tightly sealed containers (two inches deep or less).
- Date leftovers so you know how long they've been in the fridge. You can use masking tape and a sharpie to write the name of the dish and the date it was made.
- As a general rule of thumb, discard cooked leftovers after four days.
- Make it a weekly habit to throw out expired foods that should no longer be eaten.

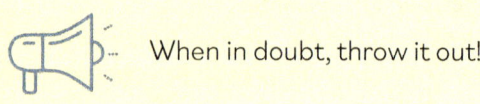 When in doubt, throw it out!

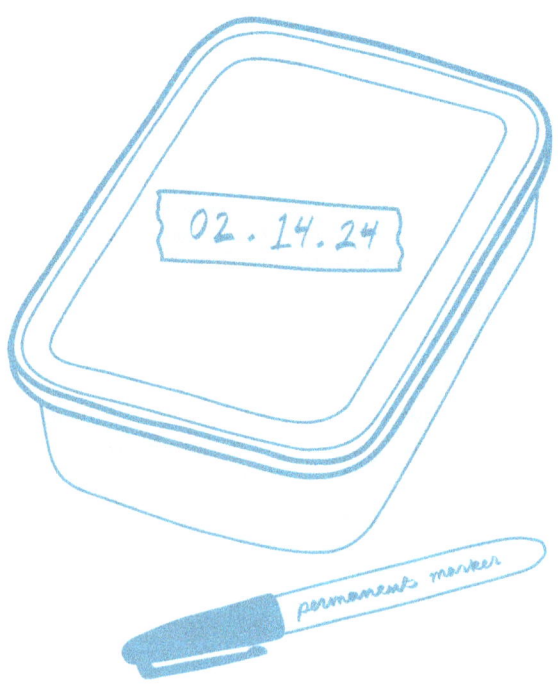

Labeled And Dated Leftovers

4. Manage Your Pantry

It's not just refrigerated food that needs attention in order to maintain good food safety practices. Proper storage and usage of dry goods (things that are boxed, bagged, canned, etc.) helps protect your food from becoming contaminated or spoiled.

Dry Goods Management

1. USE THE "FIRST IN, FIRST OUT" (FIFO) RULE
    - Food should be used in the order in which it's purchased. (Example: don't use the newest jar of spaghetti sauce first if you still have a jar from a past grocery trip.)
    - New food should be placed BEHIND the older food when you're putting groceries away.

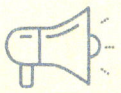

> This keeps you from finding that one random can of soup dated two years ago at the very back of the pantry.

2. PAY ATTENTION TO STORAGE TEMPERATURES
    - Just like your fridge and freezer, your pantry and dry goods storage has good and bad temperature ranges.

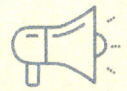

> The ideal temperature for dry goods storage is between 50°F and 70°F.

    - With each increase of 18°F, the storage life of dry goods can be cut by as much as half.

- Cool storage reduces degradation (breaking down) of food.
- Your dry goods storage should not have refrigerant units, steam/water pipes, transformers, water heaters, or other heat-producing equipment.
- Keep that pantry door closed! (You can tell your kids The Safety Queen said it's a requirement.)

3. AVOID SUNLIGHT

- Optimally, dry storage areas should NOT have windows, as sunshine can change the temperature and promote oxidation.
- If your dry goods storage has windows, it's best to block them with UV-filtering shades or blackout curtains. I know, a window in a pantry is very charming, but it's not good for your food storage.

4. KEEP THINGS OFF THE FLOOR

- All items in a pantry should be stored at least six inches off the floor. This reduces the impact from condensation that can develop with a change in temperature.
- Try to keep some distance between the top shelf and the ceiling. I know it's tempting to stack cereal boxes up to the roof and stash the stuff you don't want your family to find, but the temperature can increase as you get closer to the ceiling.

5. MANAGE PESTS AND VERMIN

- Another reason to keep stored goods off the floor is to avoid pests.
- Your boxed goods can come into your home already harboring pests like pantry moths and meal worms. If you suspect an infestation, take care of it IMMEDIATELY. How do you know if you have one? A sudden increase in moths flying around your kitchen is a common indication.

- If you have an infestation, you'll need to remove everything from your pantry. You'll likely need to throw most of it away. Wipe down every bit of the pantry with soap and water, including any shelving and plastic containers.
- Forestall any further infestations by using pantry moth traps and checking/changing them regularly.
- In some parts of the world, pantry pests are just a fact of life, and it's more about management than total elimination.

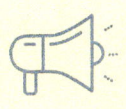

Pantry pests, much like elementary school lice, are not a reflection of your personal worthiness. Try not to let an infestation destroy your self-esteem.

6. SAFELY THROW OUT INFESTED/DAMAGED GOODS

- Very rarely, canned foods can contain bacteria known as Clostridium botulinum (we usually just call this by the toxin it creates, botulism), and consuming any contaminated food can lead to paralysis or death.
- Botulism typically comes from home-canned goods and only rarely from commercially-produced food.

NEVER eat from cans that are bulging, dented, cracked, or leaking.

- Other signs of contamination in pantry items include broken seals, corrosion, and food that looks unappealing (i.e., cloudy, moldy, disintegrating).

- Goods like flour, sugar, baking soda, etc., can also go bad. These products do have expiration dates on their packaging, but the best way to tell if they've gone bad is to smell them. If they smell "off" or "stale" or have picked up the smell of other products, throw them out. Flour that comes into contact with moisture can develop mold.

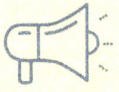 Did you know even boxed pancake and cake mixes can go bad? Typically, the baking soda in them will expire. If used, they won't perform as expected and may taste bitter.

- Properly dispose of ANY suspect food by double-bagging it and taking it straight to an outside trash can.

5. "Is This Still Good?"

We've included the most common types of food you might have in your home. These times are based on best practices.

Raw Foods	
Bacon	7 days
Chicken or turkey parts or whole	1-2 days
Eggs, fresh, in shell	3-5 weeks
Eggs, raw yolks, whites	2-4 days
Egg substitutes, liquid pasteurized eggs	Unopened, 10 days; Opened, 3 days
Fresh fish and shellfish	1-2 days
Giblets	1-2 days
Ground beef, lamb, pork, turkey, veal	1-2 days
Stew meats	1-2 days raw
Steaks, chops, roasts	3-5 days
Sausage, raw from meat or poultry	1-2 days
Variety meats (chitterlings, heart, kidneys, liver, tongue)	1-2 days

Cooked Foods	
Bacon	7 days
Beans	3-5 days
Chicken or turkey, parts or whole	3-4 days
Corned beef in pouch with pickling juices	5-7 days
Eggs, hard-cooked	1 week
Egg dishes	3-4 days
Giblets	3-4 days
Ground beef, lamb, pork, turkey, veal	3-4 days
Smoked breakfast links, patties	1-2 days
Stew meats	3-4 days
Steaks, chops, roasts	3-5 days
Ham, canned, labeled "keep refrigerated"	Unopened, 6-9 months; Opened, 3-5 days
Ham, fully cooked, sliced	3-4 days
Ham, fully cooked, halved	3-5 days
Ham, fully cooked, whole	7 days
Hard sausage (such as pepperoni)	2-3 weeks

Cooked Foods

Hot dogs	Unopened package, 2 weeks; Opened package, 1 week
Luncheon meats	Unopened package, 2 weeks; Opened package, 3-5 days
Rice, cooked	4-6 days
Soups and stews	3-4 days
Summer sausage labeled "keep refrigerated"	Unopened, 3 months; Opened, 3 weeks
Variety meats (chitterlings, heart, kidneys, liver, tongue)	3-4 days
Vegetables, cooked (in general, some have different times)	3-4 days

For downloadable versions of these tables, visit https://h2c.ai/cc.

For exhaustive lists, please visit USDA Refrigeration and Food Safety.[1]

---

[1] www.fsis.usda.gov/food-safety/safe-food-handling-and-preparation/food-safety-basics/refrigeration

6. Recalled Food Product

Food recalls can be scary if you've purchased the same or similar products.

A food recall happens when a commercial food producer has reason to believe a food item may cause illness. Recalls can happen for a variety of reasons: discovery of organisms, discovery of foreign objects such as broken glass or metal, or discovery of an allergen that doesn't appear on the label.

 A recalled food product can contaminate your kitchen, refrigerator shelves/bins, or any product it comes into contact with.

Handle Recalled Food Product

1. PHYSICALLY SEPARATE THE PRODUCT

    Include any open containers, leftover product, and anything that was prepared with the product.

2. IF THE PRODUCT HAS NEVER BEEN SERVED:

    - Throw it away, or return it for a refund if safe to do so.
    - Recall notices will often include instructions for proper disposal of the product.

3. IF THE PRODUCT INCLUDES AN ALLERGEN:

    - If the allergen is a risk for anyone in your home, throw it away, doubling your trash bags.
    - Thoroughly wash your hands before touching anything else.

4. WASH AND SANITIZE ALL COOKWARE, UTENSILS, AND CUTTING BOARDS

   See "Handwashing Dishes, Pots, Pans, and Cooking Utensils" on page 15

5. WASH AND SANITIZE ALL COUNTERTOPS AND THE INSIDE OF YOUR FRIDGE

   Reference "Sanitizing Countertops and Other Surfaces" on page 16.

WHERE TO FIND RECALL INFORMATION

The USDA maintains a food recall system. Please visit USDA Recalls and Public Health Alerts.

Top Tips for Cooking Clean

1   **MAINTAIN GOOD PERSONAL HYGIENE.**
Wash your hands, take off your jewelry, tie back your hair, and make sure any open wounds are covered. Don't prepare food if you're sick.

2   **KEEP A SANITIZED KITCHEN.**
Avoid cross-contamination. Handwash properly. Sanitize your surfaces regularly.

3   **TREAT YOUR FOOD RIGHT.**
Thaw food responsibly. Heat food up to the right temperature for each type of food. (Avoid the 100 degrees of doom!) Store it properly.

4   **MANAGE YOUR PANTRY.**
Follow FIFO. Keep food off the ground.

5   **KNOW HOW LONG YOUR FOOD IS GOOD FOR.**
Always date your leftovers. Stay on top of the inventory.

6   **HANDLE FOOD RECALLS RESONSIBLY.**
Separate and throw away any recalled food. Sanitize your kitchen.

Wrap Up & Resources

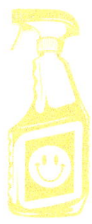 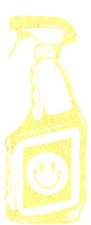 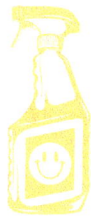

Resources

- **When and How to Clean and Disinfect Your Home**
  Centers for Disease Control and Prevention
  https://www.cdc.gov/hygiene/cleaning/cleaning-your-home.html
- **Food Safety at Home**
  U.S. Food and Drug Administration
  https://www.fda.gov/consumers/free-publications-women/food-safety-home
- **Four Steps to Food Safety: Clean, Separate, Cook, Chill**
  Centers for Disease Control and Prevention
  https://www.cdc.gov/foodsafety/communication/food-safety-in-the-kitchen.html
- **FoodSafety.gov**
  U.S. Department of Health and Human Services
  https://www.foodsafety.gov/
- **Refrigeration & Food Safety**
  United States Department of Agriculture
  https://www.fsis.usda.gov/food-safety/safe-food-handling-and-preparation/food-safety-basics/refrigeration
- **Recalls & Public Health Alerts**
  United States Department of Agriculture
  https://www.fsis.usda.gov/recalls

About the Expert

Michelle Newcome

I learned many of these basics as the person in charge of operations for a restaurant system. Done correctly and with the right attention to some basics, any home cook can build the same attention to food safety as the finest chefs do in their kitchens.

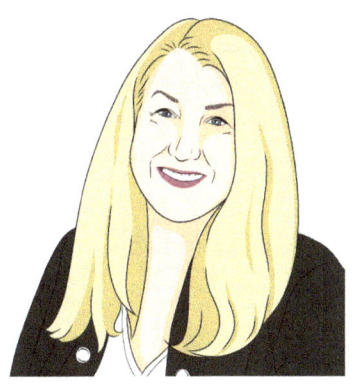

Michelle Newcome

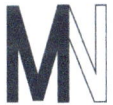 Business Resiliency Consultant | Founder and CEO of White Deer Group | Publisher of How2Conquer, imprint of White Deer Publishing, LLC

Follow Michelle on Facebook @thesafetyqueen and Instagram @MichelleConquers

About How2Conquer Guides

How2Conquer Guides are concise, approachable, and easily digestible booklets for niche subjects. With guidance from seasoned experts who don't have the time to wax poetic on their proficiency, we help connect readers with the crucial, need-to-know information that would otherwise live in the minds of the highly busy.

Find out more about our guides at how2conquer.com.

www.ingramcontent.com/pod-product-compliance
Lightning Source LLC
Chambersburg PA
CBHW052127070526
44586CB00016B/2121